෨BECOMING

by

MARTIN FAULKS

A systematic course of stretching and posture
leading to the safe and comfortable adoption of the
Lotus Posture, including a guide to the symbolism
and spiritual meaning behind the Lotus Flower

2009
Merkur Publishing, Inc.

Edited by Franca Gallo
Illustrations by Pip Faulks

Legal Notice
Please consult a doctor before performing any of the exercises in this book. The reader undertakes all exercises at his own risk. Use of this course constitutes a covenant not to bring any lawsuit or action for injury caused by performing exercises illustrated in this course. As with any form of physical exercise it is wise to seek an experienced teacher.

First Edition 2007
Second Edition 2009
ISBN 978-1885928-18-4

Published by Merkur Publishing, Inc.
PO Box 171306
Salt Lake City, UT
USA 84117
www.merkurpublishing.com

Table of Contents

The Symbolism of the Lotus Flower

The basic symbolism of the Lotus is based on the fact that the Lotus flower grows up from the mud into an object of great beauty. The Lotus flower starts its life as a bulb down at the bottom of a pond in the muck and dirt. It slowly but continually moves towards the light as it approaches the water's surface. Once it comes to the surface of the water the Lotus blooms into a beautiful flower. Indeed, in a way, as all living things come from the earth, the Lotus flower could represent life in general. In spiritual paths where the aim is to grow and change into something more beautiful and noble, this symbol represents the struggle for self-transformation perfectly.

The Lotus seed already has within itself perfectly formed embryos containing everything it needs to grow, flourish, and transform. In fact, it is said that if opened the seed even contains leaves and what appear to be whole miniature plants and flowers. This symbolises the fact that the key to our own enlightenment lies hidden within ourselves, and that nothing external is needed. On a cosmic scale this also points to the creation of the universe and the eternal great solar cycle that maintains the whole of life on earth. It also points to the ideal or spiritual world hidden within the material and the ability to access the former through the latter. Moreover, because it has buds, blossoms, and seed pods simultaneously on the same plant, it also symbolises the past, present, and future together as one.

However, the most important and powerful meaning behind the Lotus stems from the plant's mysterious ability to remain pure and unsullied. The petals reject any mud or water splashed on them and remain bright and pure. This quality of being able to remain pure when surrounded by swamp is just what the great spiritual masters of old felt was needed in an individual. If we could cultivate the ability to be unaffected by the negative things around us, then, like the lotus with its lovely scent and beautiful appearance, we could have a positive effect on the world around us.

The Universal Nature of the Lotus Symbolism

The Lotus flower has deep-rooted symbolism in every major spiritual tradition of the ancient world. We find the Lotus revered in ancient Egypt, India, Japan, and China. The Lotus ornament is also found in Assyrian, Syrian, and Carthaginian temple friezes and capitals. Indeed, it seems that wherever this plant grows, humans notice something special about it and hold it as a symbol of spiritual evolution. Although some aspects of the symbolism are constant in all these traditions, the significance of the meaning of the flower does vary slightly from one tradition to another.

Ancient Egypt

The Ancient Egyptians were fascinated by how the Lotus responded to the sun, submerging itself at night and rising above water at the break of day. To the ancient Egyptian mind, the flower was worshiping the sun and because it moved in time with the sun, disappearing and rising when it did, this meant that the Lotus was "at one" with both the sun and with the divine order of the universe (*ma-at*). In addition to the above, the Egyptians prayed each morning by burning incense, the idea being that the sweet smell would float up to the gods carrying the prayers. When the Lotus opened its petals in the morning, the sweet scent was released. To the Egyptians it was as if the Lotus was burning incense and performing its morning prayers.

So revered was this plant that Egyptian priests had their own Lotus gardens where they watched the daily re-enactment of creation's first sunrise. They concluded that the Lotus, like man and unlike the rest of the plant kingdom, responds to the presence or absence of light and warmth and this meant that it must be alive in a special way. This sun-worshiping routine made the Lotus a symbol for *Horus*, the Egyptian god of death and rebirth, and his father *Ra*, the sun god, who was born of the waters of creation each day.

In Egyptian Cosmology, the sun god *Ra* rose in the blue Lotus from *Nun*, the waters of chaos. Hidden in the Lotus' enclosing petals, as they opened, his rays of light shone bringing life and order to the universe.

The Egyptian Book of the Dead, 1240 BC (The Papyrus of *Ani*), says of the Lotus:

"As if I'd slept a thousand years underwater I wake into a new season. I am the blue lotus rising. I am the cup of dreams and memory opening — I, the thousand-petaled flower. At dawn the sun rises naked and new as a babe; I open myself and am entered by light. This is the joy, the slow awakening into fire, as one by one the petals open, as the fingers that held tight the secret unfurl. I let go of the past and release the fragrance of flowers.

"I open and light descends, fills me, and passes through, each thin blue petal reflected perfectly in clear water. I am that lotus filled with light, reflected in the world. I float content within myself, one flower with a thousand petals, one life lived a thousand years without haste, one universe sparking a thousand stars, one god alive in a thousand people.

"If you stood on a summer's morning on the bank under a brilliant sky, you would see the thousand petals and say that together they make the lotus. But if you lived in its heart, invisible from without, you might see how the ecstasy at its fragrant core gives rise to its thousand petals. What is beautiful is always that which is itself in essence, a certainty of being. I marvel at myself and the things of the earth.

"I float among the days in peace, content. Not part of the world, the world is all the parts of me. I open toward the light and lift myself to the gods on the perfume of prayer. I ask for nothing beyond myself. I own everything I need. I am content in the company of god, a prayer that contains its own answer. I am the lotus. As if from a dream, I wake up laughing."

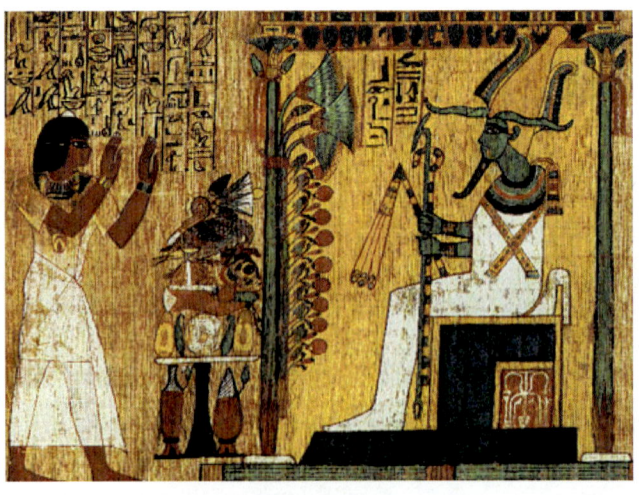

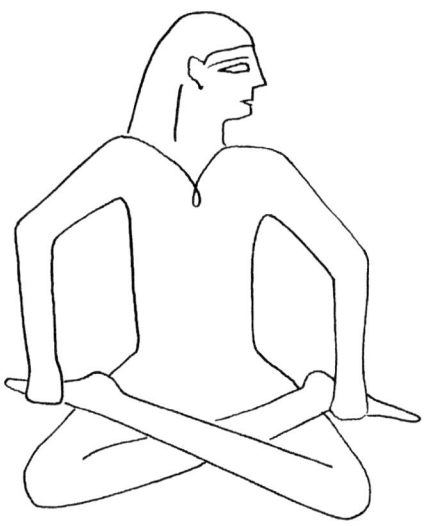

The Lotus Posture, as pictured on the walls of the tomb of
Ptah Hotep, shows that this posture has been used since the
dawn of human civilization.

Hinduism

Hindu accounts of creation state that after the utterance of
the first *Om*, the vast primordial ocean brought forth a
glorious golden Lotus, resplendent as the sun, which
floated upon the divine waters. Standing upon that *Om*
were the divine trinity of Brahma, Vishnu and Shiva. Thus
the Lotus flower is the most divine and sacred symbol of
the Hindu religion. In fact, the Hindu word for worship is
"*puja*," which translates literally as "flower act." Hindu
texts describe that water represents the procreative aspect
of the Divinity and that the golden Lotus represents the
opposite generative force, the Lotus being the first product
of the creative principle.

In another tale, the role of Lord Brahma is to re-create the universe after a great flood destroyed the whole of creation. In order to do this he uses the different parts of the Lotus plant.

It is rare to find a Hindu god who is not associated with the Lotus in some way. Indeed, virtually every God and Goddess of Hinduism — Brahma, Vishnu, Shiva, Saraswati, Durga, Ganesha, Rama and Surya, Lakshmi Agni, and Parvati are normally shown sitting on the Lotus or holding Lotus flowers. The Lotus serves thus as the seat of the Deity, signifying its divinity and purity.

According to the sacred text of the Bhagavad-Gita, man should aim to be like the Lotus — he should work without attachment, dedicating his actions to the divine. Then, like the Lotus, he will be untouched by sin just as mud has no effect on the Lotus. In Hinduism the Lotus flower also represents the awakening to the spiritual part of a man. In fact, the highest chakra on the top of the head is known as the Thousand-petaled Lotus. This is said to open when enlightenment is gained.

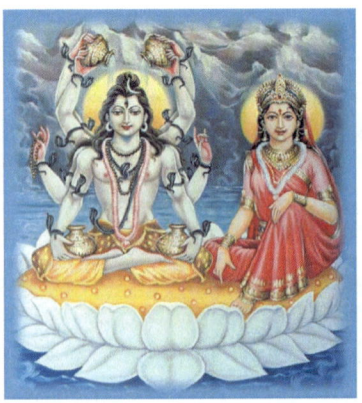

A depiction of Shiva and Shakti on a Lotus flower.

Buddhism

In Buddhism, the Lotus symbolizes man in his highest, most exalted, pure, and undefiled state — one of complete balance, his feet rooted on the ground and his face to the heavens. It is said that on the night that Gautama Buddha was conceived, a huge Lotus grew out of the earth. As one enlightened during his lifetime, Buddha is often pictured on a Lotus throne. This represents Buddha's mastery over the intellectual and philosophic world. This is that aim of all Buddhists as expressed in the Buddhist mantra *Om mani padme hum*, which translates as "The jewel at the heart of the lotus."

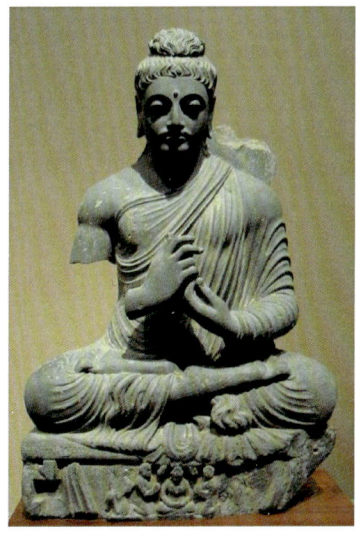

Seated Buddha, Gandhara, 1st-2nd century CE.

Christianity

The Christian equivalent of the Lotus is the white lily. This relates to the Virgin Mary as queen of heaven and represents purity, fertility, peace, chastity, and innocence. Traditionally, the Archangel Gabriel carries the lily to symbolize purity. "Blessed are the pure in heart," said Jesus, "for they shall see God."

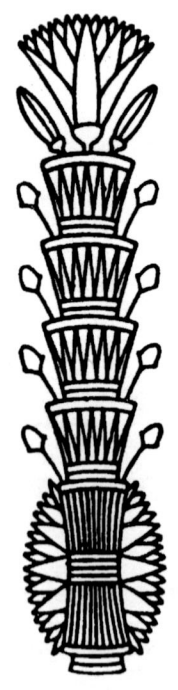

Colour Symbolism of the Lotus Flowers

White Lotus

This represents the state of total mental purity that opens the path to spiritual perfection.

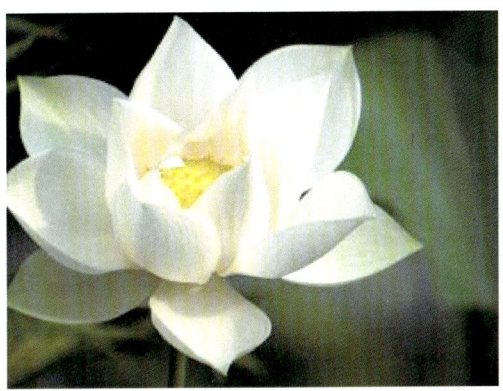

Red Lotus

This is the Lotus of love, passion, will, activity, and ambition. This symbolizes all the qualities of the heart. This Lotus is normally represented with its petals closed.

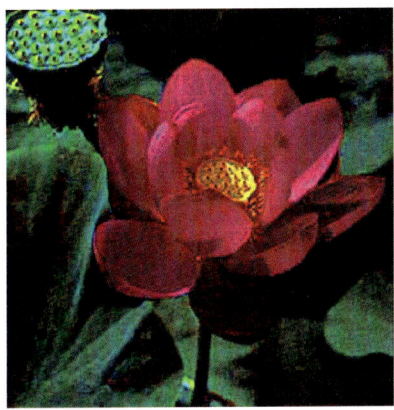

Blue Lotus

This is the symbol of the victory of the spirit over the material world. It symbolises the development of wisdom and spiritual powers that allow you to sense the spiritual world. This Lotus is normally represented with its petals closed.

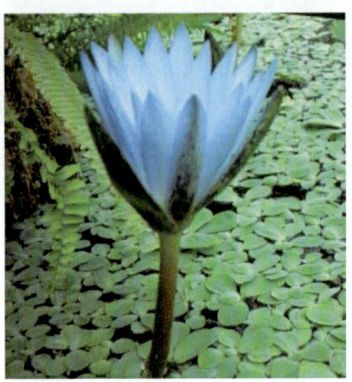

Pink Lotus

This is the supreme lotus, representing the attainment of deity status.

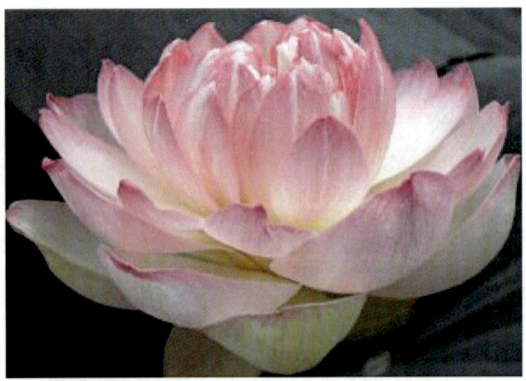

Purple Lotus

The most mystic Lotus, only represented in the images belonging to a few esoteric sects, its meaning is shrouded and known only by the select few.

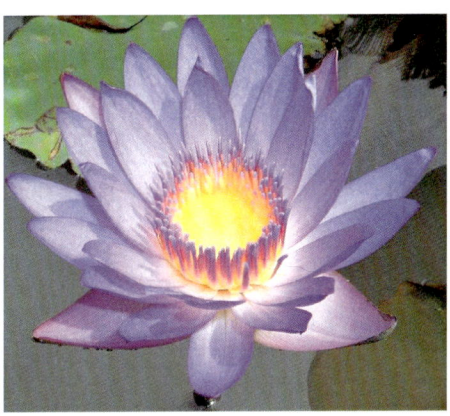

About the Lotus, Botanically Speaking

The Lotus plant is an aquatic perennial with the botanical name of *Nelumbo Nucifera*, though it has many variants and grows in many different colours varying from white to blue, yellow, and even bright pink.

Each variety has a different Latin name. For example, the sacred blue Lotus depicted in the Egyptian *Book of the Dead* with its beautiful pointed petals that used to grow on the banks of the River Nile is called *Nymphaea Caerulea*. A once common flower in ancient times, the Lotus is almost extinct in the wilds of Africa. However, it is still quite common in many Asian countries.

Most of the plant is edible and the petals are often used as a garnish. The leaves can be used like vine leaves to wrap food. In China the roots, stalk, petals, and leaves are often stir-fried or even eaten raw. The Lotus seeds are often made into flour or popped like popcorn! The stamens make a lovely fragrant, calming tea. You must try it if you are ever in China.

The Lotus Posture

Accepted throughout the world as the best posture for meditation and contemplation, the yoga posture is the only seated pose in which all four areas of the body are perfectly balanced, the legs and feet, pelvis and torso, the arms and hands, the neck, throat, and head are all in perfect alignment. When the body is in perfect balance so is the spirit; the head rests correctly on the spinal column and breathing becomes easy. The positioning of the legs in the Lotus Posture supports the back and aligns the torso so the diaphragm is able to expand more fully.

The locking of the legs together also provides a solid foundation, a base on which you feel secure and stable. In the Lotus Posture you feel firmly connected to the earth and yet your mind is clear and alert.

One Indian text, the Yoga-Shastra, even describes 840,000 different yoga poses, but only describes the Lotus Posture (*Padmasana*) as suitable for attaining enlightenment.

Become a Lotus in your Innermost First

The Lotus Posture is without doubt the supreme position for meditation. The problem is that many people trying to sit in the position have not learned to become like the

Lotus in their innermost first. They are too influenced by wanting to rush and impress people. Unlike the Lotus the outside world is affecting them and they are being motivated by ego. Before you become the Lotus in posture you really need to be like the Lotus in your spirit. You need to be calm and patient. You should let yourself progress at a natural calm rate without rushing or worrying about how long it is going to take you. It is not important how long it takes you. The important thing is that like the Lotus you grow steadily towards your goal without letting any frustration or setback upset you or affect what you are doing. If you follow this course properly you should be able to sit in the Lotus position within a year, probably sooner. We are, however, all individuals and progress at our own rate. It is far better to take your time and progress without haste than to rush, force your body and cause injury. Becoming the Lotus is really the lesson that the posture teaches — be sure to make the inner change your focus as much as the outer ability to do the posture. This is the only way you will make satisfactory progress.

Why You Need this Course

There is a great danger of knee damage connected with the Lotus Posture. This is caused when people with insufficient hip flexibility try to force him- or herself into the position too early. The only way to protect the knees in the Lotus Posture (in all its variations) is to follow a systematic course in hip flexibility such as the one outlined here. Then and only then will you be able to achieve the Lotus position in comfort and safety. People are continually injuring their knees through the Lotus Posture — forcing one's legs into the Lotus Posture is painful. That feeling of pain is your knees telling you not to do it. Pain is an important warning sign that you should never ignore. If your teacher or instructor tries to force you to perform this or any posture through pain, you should leave his or her tutorage. You will not achieve enlightenment with this method; you will achieve a painful pinching sensation in the inner knee that will lead to injury. If you are using your knees to flex into the Lotus position you are pinching the inner cartilage of the knee between the inner ends of the thigh and shin bones, while simultaneously over-stretching the tendon on the outside of the knee.

Incorrect Lotus Posture Diagram

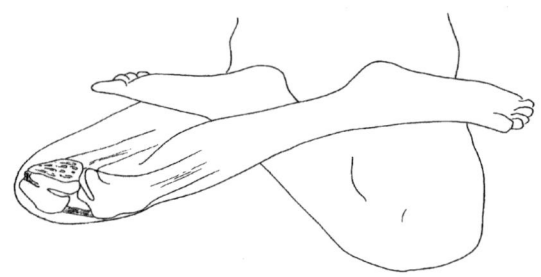

Notice in the above diagram —

> ➤ The stretch comes from the knee, not the hip.
> ➤ The feet face upwards.
> ➤ The cartilage on one side of the knee joint is crushed.
> ➤ The lateral collateral ligament near the bottom on the knee is being overstretched.

Here is an easy exercise to help you discover if you are doing the Lotus position correctly.

Sit with both feet facing forward. Bend your right leg at the knee. Now rotate your hips so that your knee moves in a rightward, downward arch towards the floor. Keep going until you can't go any further. If you can rotate your hip enough to get your foot up on your opposite thigh you are doing fine. This requires continuing to rotate the hip even after the right knee has touched the floor. If you can't manage this movement and have to lift the foot and stretch from the knee after your hip stops externally rotating, you are doing the pose incorrectly.

How to Perform the Lotus Posture Correctly

The Lotus Posture requires a great deal of hip flexibility. To get into this posture safely the head of the thighbone must rotate outward in the hip socket about $120°$. If your hips are this flexible you can sit in the Lotus position correctly. Then you can leave your knees to just bend forwards and back like they were designed for!

This course is going to show you how to increase the flexibility in your hip joints and to build strength in the muscles around them, so you can do the Lotus Posture the correct way.

But this is going to take a while. In our culture our hips have adapted to our sitting on chairs rather than sitting on the floor. A lifetime of prolonged sitting on chairs causes shortening of the very muscles and ligaments needed to be flexible in the Lotus Posture.

The hip is a ball-and-socket joint with some of the strongest ligaments in the body to keep it stable. This in turn leads to it being very hard to increase flexibility in this joint. The only way to make any progress is through gentle and persistent ongoing practice.

Correct Lotus Posture Diagram

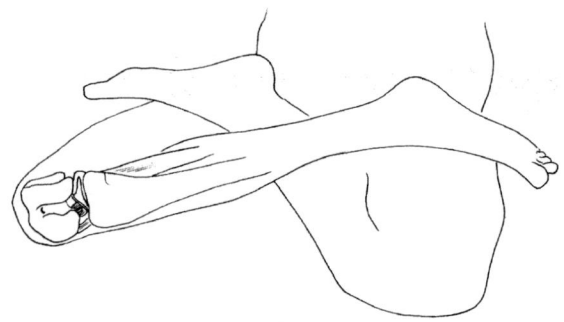

Notice in the above diagram —

> ➤ The stretch comes from the hip not the knee.
> ➤ The feet face backwards.
> ➤ The knee is in healthy alignment.

How to Perform the Stretches

The following series will lead you into the Lotus Posture in a safe and comfortable way. The stretches are best done after the body is warmed up either through other exercise or through the optional "crow walking" exercise described in this volume. You will find that you are more flexible in the evening than you are in the morning. It is recommended that the exercises be performed twice a day. If performed before any formal meditation these exercises will improve the quality of your sitting no matter what position you are currently using. You will also learn other postures that are of great benefit to you.

Begin by holding each position for one minute, then increase to three minutes as the pose becomes easier. It is a good idea to use a timer for consistency as it is difficult to know how long you are in a posture without one and your mood will dictate your posture timing too much.

Use deep abdominal breathing in all stretches and relax your body as you exhale. Let your body relax into the posture rather than pressing the muscles into the stretch. Mentally welcome the posture and let the body progress at its own rate. Let the posture and the body meet on their own terms, in their own time. If you force the body, you may set up a conflicting relationship between what you think your body *should* be capable of and what the body *is* capable of. You will start to view your body as an enemy to be defeated rather than a companion on the journey. Practice without expectation — that way even a difficult pose will become easy and enjoyable, and you will progress quickly toward achievement of the Lotus Posture.

Remember: You should feel a slight stretch but never any discomfort or pain.

Stretching Postures
The Crow Walking Pose (optional warm-up)

This is a wonderful exercise to warm your legs up before you perform any of the stretching exercises or before any seated meditation posture.

Performance:
> Stand with your feet shoulder width apart. Squat down so your buttocks touch your heels. Place your hands on your knees. Keep your back straight. This is your ready position.
>
> Begin taking small steps while still squatting. Be careful to keep your balance. Keep the knees bent throughout the movement. With time and practice you will be able to increase the length of your steps so that you can move through a full range of movements, putting one knee next to the opposite knee with each step. This is a great warm-up move for the hips as you can simply take steps until you are warmed up, but it is best avoided if you have any knee problems.

Benefits
> • Best warm-up for legs prior to sitting for meditation;
> • Improves circulation in legs;
> • Can relieve constipation.

Contraindications
> • Avoid crow walking while you have any toe, ankle, or especially knee complaints.

Hints
- Make the walking smooth and even. Note the sensations in your hips, legs, and lower back afterwards. Avoid going more than forty to fifty steps.

Lotus Lunge 1
(also known as "The Pigeon" in Yoga)

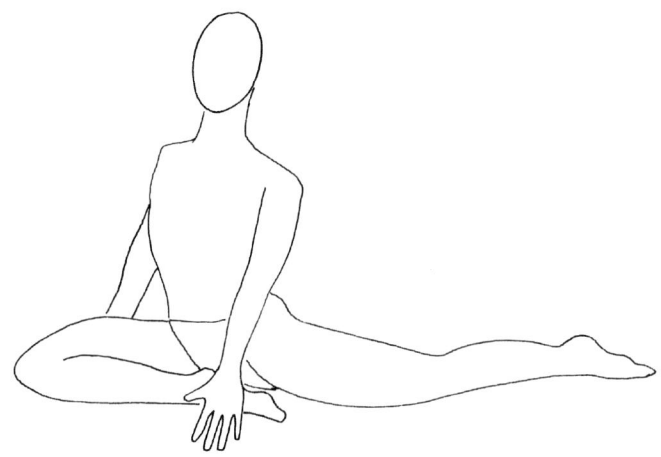

This is perhaps the most important exercise of the whole course. It gives your hips the specific stretch that you should feel in many of the other exercises and has a direct effect on the directional flexibility needed for the Lotus Posture. It is a bit awkward to start with, so you really should ensure you have mastered the technique for this exercise before moving onto the next level.

Performance:
Stand with your feet about shoulder width apart. Bend your knees and squat down keeping your back straight. Place your hands on the floor so as to support the weight of your body. Extend the left leg out behind

you, the top of the foot touching the floor and the kneecap facing downward. Then rotate the bent right leg so that the knee moves outwards and bring the heel of the right foot to the pubic bone. Keep your torso lifted and as upright as possible. Feel the stretch on the buttock of the right leg. Repeat on the other side.

Lotus Lunge 2

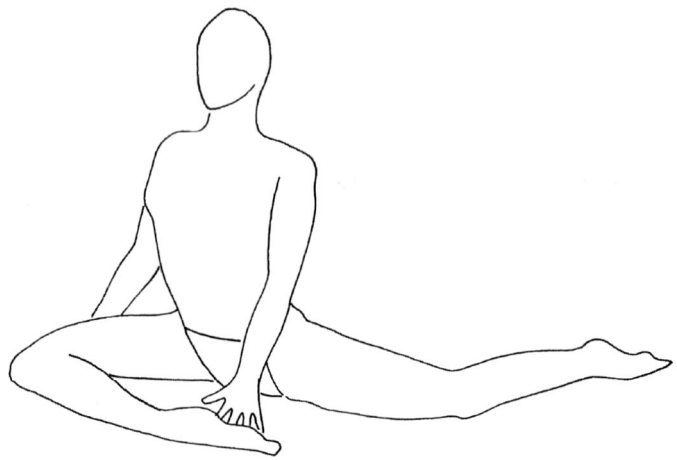

To add to the intensity of this stretch, unbend the leading leg slightly so that the foot moves away from the thigh. Open the leg to an angle of about 45°, being careful to stretch from the hip, not the knee. Repeat on the other side.

Benefits
- Improves hip flexibility in two directions as your rear leg is stretched backwards and your front leg is given a rotational stretch;
- Improves circulation in the pelvic area;
- Said to increase energy and vitality;

- Gives mild stretch to the back and neck helping to remove backache and fatigue;
- Makes legs appear long and shapely;
- Helps shoulder strength.

Contraindications
- Beware of overloading the knee or hip as you lower weight;
- Avoid if you have unhealthy knees;
- Practice gently if you have a slipped disc.

Hints
- Try also letting the front leg find its position naturally as you lower yourself. Beware of cheating by over flexing the spine just above the pelvis.

The Cradle Stretch

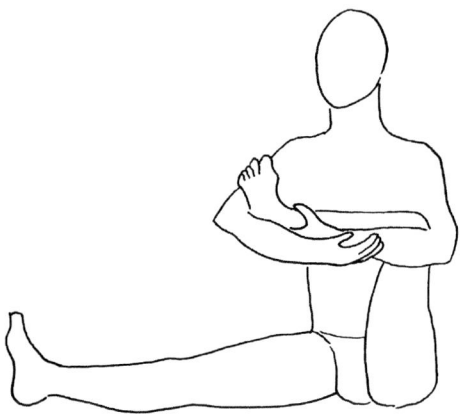

Sit with both your legs straight out before you. Bend your right knee and rotate your leg out. Put the sole of the right foot in the crease of the left elbow and hold the knee in the crease of the right elbow. Clasp your hands together. Now rotate the hip so that you are holding your leg in your arms as you would a baby. To increase the stretch keep moving the right foot away from the floor. You may also hug the leg towards your chest slightly, but be careful not to stretch from the knee. Repeat on the other side.

Benefits
- Increases blood supply to the hip;
- Increases flexibility through the hip and glutes;
- Gently massages abdomen, so helps digestion.

Contraindications
- None.

Hints
- Avoid torso movement to isolate the effect.

Through the Hole Stretch

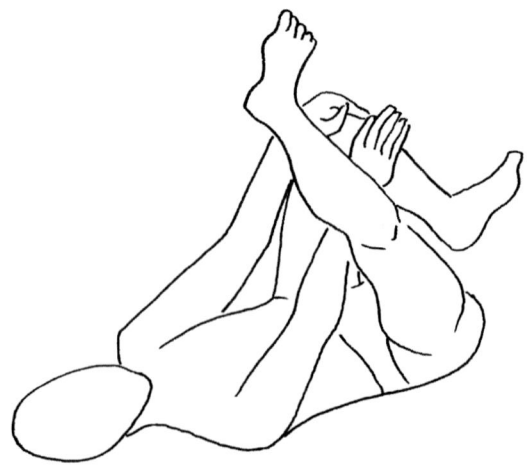

Lie down and bend both knees. Cross your right leg over the left placing the foot so the calf is resting on the left thigh. Take the right arm through the gap of the right leg around the back of the left thigh. Clasp your hands. As you draw the left thigh toward you, turn the right hip out and move the right knee away from you to open the hip. Repeat on the other side.

Benefits
- Improves hip flexibility;
- Stretches adductors;
- Stretches deep back muscles;
- As the spine is stable this is very safe;
- Some toning of ascending and descending colon.

Contraindications
- Avoid if knees are unhealthy;
- If pregnant, avoid after the first trimester.

Hints
- When lifting legs the pelvis may lift. This is acceptable, but to increase the efficiency of this stretch isometrically push it back toward the floor;
- Also try varying where you hold the leg, sometimes through the hole, sometimes above it.

Head to Knee Posture 1

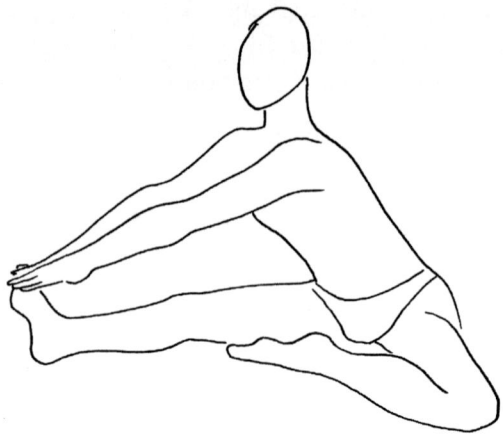

Sit with both legs straight before you. Bend your left knee and rotate the left thigh out as far as possible placing your left foot next to your right thigh. Turn your body to face towards the big toe of the extended right leg. Reach for your right knee and bend forward from the hips over the right leg. Repeat with the positions of the legs reversed.

Head to Knee Posture 2

This stretch is the more advanced form of the former exercise and is performed identically to the above, except in this case instead of placing the foot of the bent leg next to the thigh of the other leg, you lift your left leg into the Cradle Stretch (as illustrated on pages 25-26), and then gently place your left ankle on top of the right thigh so that the heel touches your lower abdomen or as close to your abdomen as you can get. Do not worry if you cannot touch the floor with the left knee. In time, as your flexibility increases, you will find that your knee moves with increasing ease toward the floor.

Benefits
- Stretches the hamstrings;
- Increases hip flexibility;
- Helps urinary function;
- As you get lower it also massages your entire abdomen, improving organ function;
- Has been said to help control diabetes;
- Improves spine condition;
- Helps relieve constipation.

Contraindications
- Avoid if you have a slipped disc or sciatica.

Hints
- After practicing this exercise it is good to realign the knee by sitting with your feet out in front and lifting the leg with the hands just above the knee whilst pulling your foot back towards the shin. Do both sides.

Leg Behind Arm Stretch

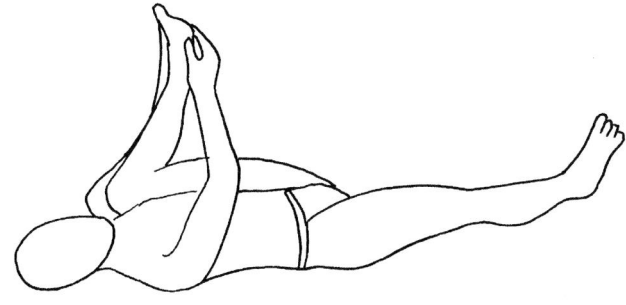

Lie on your back with the legs straight. Bend your left knee and hold the foot with both hands. Move the knee down towards the floor past your rib cage. Keep the left leg down flat on the floor. Repeat on the other side.

Benefits
- Improves flexibility of adductors;
- Can help digestive function.

Contraindications
- Not for those with severe back problems, e.g. slipped disc.

Hints
- Avoid tilting sideways with leg raised. Try co-ordinating breath by exhaling as you move the thigh down. Be careful as your shoulders can pull harder than your hips can resist. You can also do both legs at once.

The Graceful Seat Pose

Start by kneeling on the floor. Have your knees/legs hip-width apart so that the thighs are parallel with one an-other; separate your legs so they are slightly wider than your hips. Ensure that your knees keep facing downwards and that your feet still face towards the floor.

Sit between your feet by supporting yourself with your hands and then slowly lowering your buttocks to the floor until you feel a stretch.

After a while you will be able to sit in this position with your buttocks planted firmly on the ground. Use your arms for support until you can hold this position with ease. It may take several months until you can achieve this.

Benefits
- Helps prevent hernia;
- Helps relieve piles;
- Can help remove stomach disorders;
- Helps genitals.

Contraindications
- Avoid if knees are unhealthy.

Hints
- One should never strain with this pose;
- Experiment with a blanket folded to the point where you can lower to and so rest upon it. This stimulates the perineum which in turns relaxes the nervous system.

Reclining Graceful Seat Pose

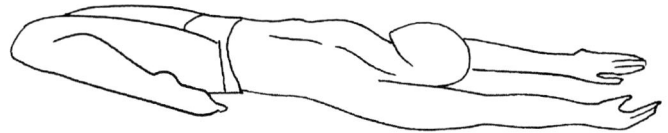

Sit in the Graceful Seat Pose as normal; recline backwards, resting on your elbows. Go as far as is comfortable depending on your flexibility, your aim being to eventually recline on the floor with the arms over the head. Do not attempt to recline if the knees splay out or lift off the floor. The stretch should be done with the knees facing the floor.

Benefits
- Realigns rounded shoulders;
- Tones the spine;
- Helps breathing, i.e. can relieve asthma, bronchitis etc.;
- Loosens legs prior to meditation;
- Great abdominal stretch when the arms are above the head.

Contraindications
- This pose is also not intended for those who have back problems;
- Also avoid this pose if pregnant.

Angled Splits Stretch

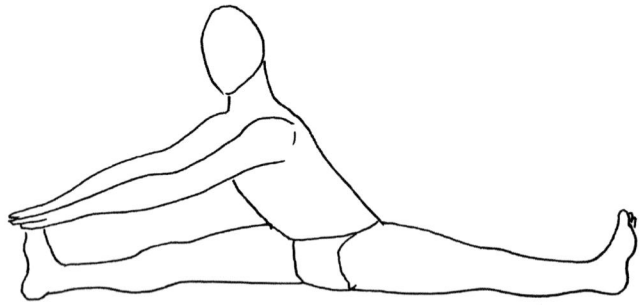

Sit with your legs spread as wide apart as you can. You should feel a slight stretch in your inner thighs. Turn and bend your torso towards your thigh and reach for the right toe. Repeat on the other side.

Benefits
- Gives good stretch to adductors;
- Increases flexibility and circulation in pelvic region;

- Improves hamstring flexibility;
- Makes legs appear long and shapely.

Contraindications
  - Practice only gently if any back ailments exist.

Hints
  - As you are able to move further towards your toes, and out even beyond them you can also try stretching out forwards. As your splits get wider you can reach a point where the thighs are out of the way of the pelvis and you can lean (with a straight back) until your front, including the pelvis, lies on the floor. If you can do this, the Lotus Pose is well within your reach.

The Tailor's Stretch

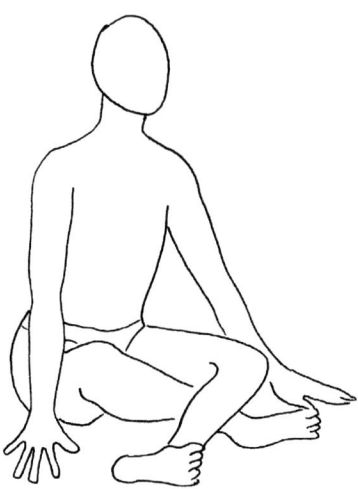

Sit on the floor with your legs crossed. Extend your legs forward and away from the groin while keeping them crossed. Keep going until your feet are at right angles. Lean forward with your back straight while supporting yourself with your arms on the floor. Feel the stretch on the outside of the hips. Repeat, changing which way round your legs are crossed.

Benefits
- Improves abductor flexibility;
- Improves digestion.

Contraindications
- Only practice mildly if you have a slipped disc.

Hints
- Avoid putting pressure on the bottom leg. Be careful to keep your back straight to ensure efficiency of the pose. It's all right to take the body's weight on your arms.

Cross-Legged Stretch

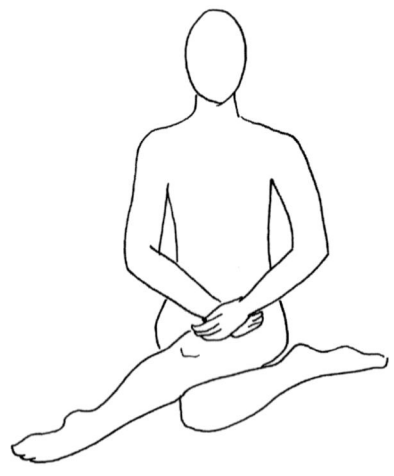

Sit with the legs extended in front of you. Cross your right leg over your left leg. Bend your knee and slide your left leg along the floor, until your left foot comes in contact with the right buttock. You may have to aid this process with your hands. Now gently guide your right heel with your hands until it touches the left buttock. The knees should rest one atop the other.

Benefits
- Massages and tones pelvic and reproductive organs.

Butterfly Knees

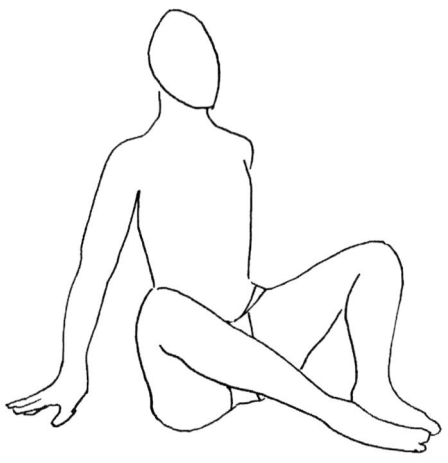

Sit with your knees bent and the soles of your feet together. Grasp your feet with your hands and pull your heels as close toward your groin as possible. Gently direct your knees towards the floor. As your knees lower to the floor it is acceptable to allow the feet to separate as if they were a book, with the sides of the feet touching the floor (being the binding) and the upper big toe side of the feet, the pages.

When your knees can reach the floor, you can use a block under the feet to help get more stretch in the inner thighs as the knees descend.

Benefits
- Rejuvenates your legs if you have been standing for a long time;
- Stretches inner thighs (adductors).

Contraindications
- Again, avoid if you have sciatica or any problem in the spine through the sacral plexus.

Lying Butterfly Knees

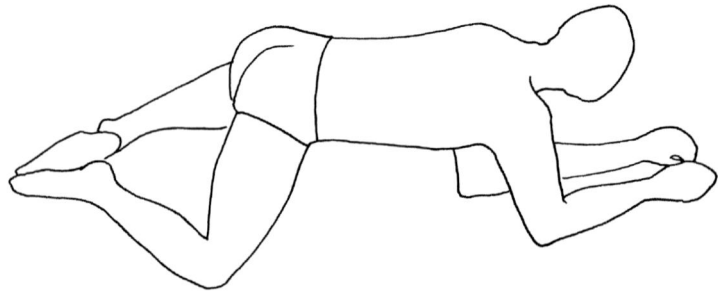

Kneel on a carpet. Lean forwards, taking your weight on your forearms. Slowly let the knees move outwards with your feet touching. Move your body slightly forwards and relax into the stretch.

Benefits
- Excellent for adductor flexibility;
- Also good for back and shoulder strength as you have to avoid slipping.

Contraindications
- Avoid this pose if you have back, shoulder, or knee problems;
- Definitely do not risk slipping if you are pregnant.

Hints
- If you really master this exercise, then instead of moving the body forward, move back gently.

Seated Postures
Use a Cushion

Do not be afraid to use props to make the sitting time more comfortable. You can use folded blankets, or a special meditation cushion (sometimes called *zafu*). This is especially good for the Lotus Posture variations as it helps keep your knees lower than your hips. However, ensure that it is a low cushion. You want to aid your knees to descend toward the floor, but you don't want to overwork the forward tilt of your pelvis.

The Burmese Posture

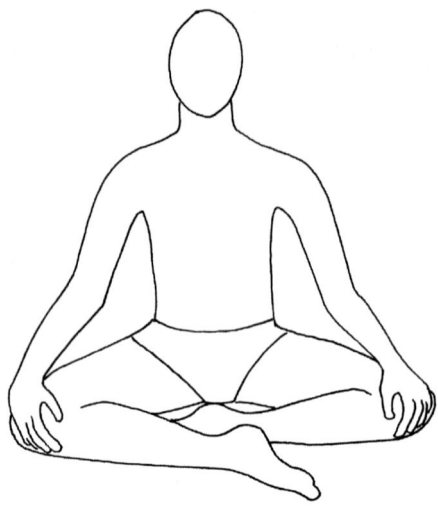

This is one of the best meditation postures in existence.
For years I was using more complicated postures and found
that after long periods my legs were numb. I also found it
annoying that often I had to meditate when travelling or
pushed for time and didn't have time to warm up. This
posture was recommended to me by a Japanese master who
informs me that this posture is very common in Zen practice. This is a simple posture to master, compared to the
Lotus, and will be of use to you for the rest of your life. It
also stretches the hips and opens them in preparation for
the Lotus Posture. In this posture the legs are not crossed,
and the knees are turned outwards to the floor. The legs
are bent and the feet placed in front of the pelvis with one
foot in front of the other. Your hands rest on top of the
thighs or on the heels. Feel free to adjust the position of
the feet until you are comfortable; it is perfectly acceptable to either have the feet straight in front of each other,

or to let them pass so that one foot is next to the other ankle. You may also have to adjust the angle to allow you to place your calves or knees on the floor.

In the Burmese Posture you must pay attention to keeping your legs on the floor. When you cross your legs in the Full or Half Lotus position, it naturally pushes the knees down. Not so with the Burmese Posture. It may take a while for you to sit comfortably in this position. To begin with you may not be able to rest your legs down comfortably; do not worry about this, for you will find that this improves as the course progresses. If you are already practicing meditation, I advise you to convert to the Burmese Posture to help prepare yourself for the Lotus Posture.

The Half Lotus Posture

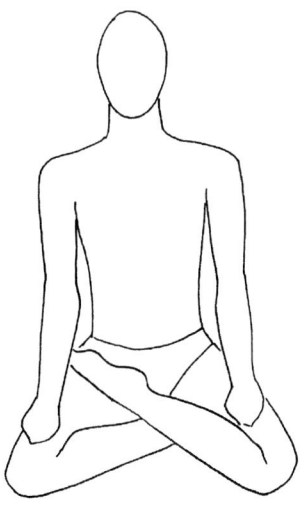

Sit in the Burmese Posture. Pick up your right foot with both hands, and bring it up into the Cradle position. Sit in a relaxed upright manner.

Place the right foot in the crease formed by the left thigh and the upper body. Adjust the left foot forward until it sits comfortably under the right knee. Now your right leg should be in a tight Half Lotus. Adjust your position so you can sit erect.

If your knee does not rest comfortably on the left foot then gently press down with your right hand. Hold the stretch 30 seconds or so and repeat. Never bounce your knee up and down. Repeat with the other leg.

Do not worry if both knees do not rest on the floor or mat. Time will remedy that at its own pace.

The Full Lotus Posture

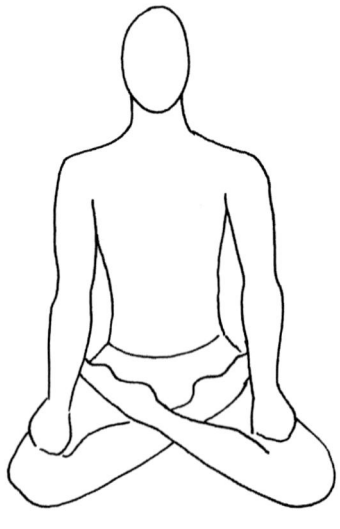

Sit with your legs straight out before you. Sit on a cushion or folded mat to elevate the hips and allow the knees to sink through hip rotation. Keeping the back upright, bring your right leg into the Cradle Stretch position and externally rotate the right hip. Keep the right foot flexed; this helps prevents rotation at the knee and ankle joints. Place the right foot on top of the left thigh.

Relax the entire right leg. Now slowly bend the left knee in towards the folded right leg. Cross the leg in front of you. Pick up your left foot and lower shin and gently lift it onto the right thigh. You have now completed the pose. The left knee may be slightly above the floor. Relax, with practice this will even up.

Sit in a balanced upright position. The ideal position is not hard to find, just watch your breathing and position yourself where it is most free and easy.

Either rest the hands on the knees with the palms facing up or hold them together on your lap. Start by staying in the pose for brief periods, increasing your stay as your hips increase in flexibility.

When your legs grow tired, stretch them straight out before you and gently massage your knees. Cross your legs the other way around and practice on the other side.

Benefits of the Lotus Pose
- Strengthens the back;
- Improves posture;
- Improves circulation between the legs and torso;
- Increases circulation in the lumbar area and the abdomen;
- Calms the mind;

- Aids digestion and peristaltic movement;
- Increases circulation to abdominal organs;
- Best meditation posture, as it provides the classical sitting position for longer periods of time without bodily movement;
- Promotes great mobility of the ankles, knees, and hips;
- Relaxes the nervous system;
- Reduces blood pressure;
- Reduces muscle and skin tension;
- Nerves in the lower back are toned by increased blood supply.

Benefits are the same but less significant in the Half Lotus and less again in the Burmese Posture.

Contraindications
- Do not practice if you have sciatica;
- Avoid if there is any infection in the sacrum;
- Just practice the Burmese Posture if your knees are injured or inflamed.

Hints
- Hip flexibility alone will not make the Lotus Pose perfect. Good back strength and certain flexibility in the knees are required. The exercises herein will provide the necessary knee flexibility. To strengthen the back, you need do only one thing. Practice! Build up slowly, sitting for longer periods. Do not go so far that your back becomes stiff or your muscles spasm. Sitting for long periods can be quite difficult. It takes practice. Just make it a habit in your daily life, when you can, to sit cross-legged on the floor with a straight back.

A Systematic Course in Stretching Leading to the Full Lotus Posture

In this chapter you will find a progressive course in stretching, leading to the Lotus Posture. This is the start of your journey towards the Lotus Posture. Your first main aim is for you to get into the habit of performing a daily stretching routine. The easiest way, as with all disciplines, is for you to perform the routine at the same time every day. Humans are creatures of habit and if you make your practice part of your daily routine it will be easier to stick to. I always stretch in the morning before my meditation. I suggest a regular practice time, which will help you too. Take a while to familiarize yourself with the postures and to ensure that you are happy with the whole process of getting in and out of each posture. Then you are ready to introduce them into your daily routine. Starting with level one, work through each routine only moving up when all the exercises come with perfect ease. Make certain that you have completely mastered one set of exercises before you proceed to the next. Let the body take its own time and enjoy the process of working steadily towards your goal.

Level 1
Daily Routine: Crow Walking (Optional), Lotus Lunge 1, Burmese Posture.

Level 2
Daily Routine: Lotus Lunge 1, Cradle Stretch, Burmese Posture.

Level 3
Daily Routine: Lotus Lunge 1, Cradle Stretch, Through the Hole Stretch, Burmese Posture.

Level 4
Daily Routine: Lotus Lunge 2, Head to Knee Posture 1, Cradle Stretch, Through the Hole Stretch, Butterfly Knees, Burmese Posture.

Level 5
Daily Routine: Lotus Lunge 2, Head to Knee Posture 2, Leg Behind Arm Stretch, Cradle Stretch, Through the Hole Stretch, Angled Splits Stretch, Reclining Graceful Seat Pose, Butterfly Knees, Burmese Posture.

Level 6
Daily Routine: Lotus Lunge 2, Head to Knee Posture 2, Leg Behind Arm Stretch, Cradle Stretch, Through the Hole Stretch, Angled Splits Stretch, Reclining Graceful Seat Pose, Butterfly Knees, Half Lotus.

Level 7
Daily Routine: Lotus Lunge 2, Head to Knee Posture 2, Leg Behind Arm Stretch, Cross-legged Stretch, Tailor's Stretch, Angled Splits Stretch, Reclining Graceful Seat Pose, Butterfly Knees, Half Lotus.

Level 8
Daily Routine: Lotus Lunge 2, Head to Knee Posture 2, Leg Behind Arm Stretch Cross-legged Stretch, Tailor's Stretch, Angled Splits Stretch, Reclining Graceful Seat Pose, Butterfly Knees, Lying Butterfly Knees, Half Lotus.

Level 9
Daily Routine: Lotus Lunge 2, Head to Knee Posture 2, Leg Behind Arm Stretch Cross-legged Stretch, Tailor's Stretch, Angled Splits Stretch, Reclining Graceful Seat Pose, Butterfly Knees, Lying Butterfly Knees, Half Lotus.

Level 10

Daily Routine: Lotus Lunge 2, Head to Knee Posture 2, Cross-legged Stretch, Tailor's Stretch, Angled Splits Stretch, Reclining Graceful Seat Pose, Butterfly Knees, Lying Butterfly Knees, Half Lotus, Full Lotus.

"Opening the Lotus Flower" Meditation

"Opening the Lotus Flower" or the "Lotus Flower Breath" is a traditional Chinese Daoist meditation technique. The aim of this meditation is to quieten your mind so that you can come into contact with the calmness and inner peace that is always deep inside you.

The regular practice of the Lotus Breath offers many benefits including: stress reduction, clearer thinking, more creative thinking, greater ability to cope, an increased sense of peace and contentment, and helps to balance the emotions. It builds the internal strength and clears the meridians, curing illness and bringing great benefit. After the first month, you will see great effects on your body, soul, and spirit. Hundreds of modern scientific studies now confirm what spiritual masters have been saying for 5,000 years. Meditation really is one of the most healthy exercises a human can practice.

As with your stretching exercises, it is best to choose a specific time or times for your meditation. I would advise that you start with 5 minutes in the morning and 5 in the evening. Then slowly work each session up to 20 minutes. Choose a nice relaxing and calming place to practice your meditation. If you always meditate in the same place, you will create an association of meditation and peacefulness with the space you have chosen. Then each time you come back to this space, you will anticipate the experience of meditation. You will also develop your own rituals that you in turn will associate with preparing to meditate, such as taking the phone off the hook or lighting incense. It is advisable to use a timer, such as an electronic timer, to monitor your meditation and to "beep" when it is time for you to stop.

How to Perform the Meditation

Sit in the Burmese Posture or the Lotus Posture. Start your meditation by focusing on your breath. Imagine that as you breathe in, you are breathing in calmness and relaxation and that with each exhalation you are breathing out tension and worry. Take time to notice how slowly each and every part of your body relaxes in its own time.

Now as you breathe in, imagine that with every breath you breathe in a glowing white light. Imagine that every pore in your body is absorbing this force with each and every breath you take. As you breathe in, this spiritual force is focused into one small glowing point in your Dantien (the centre of your body, two to three inches below your navel). With each breath this tiny bead of light grows. Imagine that it radiates health and harmony as it shines. Really imagine that with every breath you take you draw this healing force from the very limits of the universe; and with each breath imagine that you charge this point of light, which you should imagine growing in size and forming into the bud of a Lotus flower. Continue to condense this force with each breath, being careful not to extend your breathing in an unnatural manner, but rather breathing in a natural and relaxed manner. Remember, it is your mental focus that is important.

Soon when the time is right the Lotus bud will start to open in your innermost, the petals divided into shards of light. Soon your whole torso will contain this flower. When this happens a great calmness ensues. You should ensure that your mind is filled with a complete assurance that the light emitted by this spiritual Lotus heals and balances all the systems in your body. Keep your mind on this image for the remainder of the meditation. Continue to imagine that with each breath you take you feed this healing and balancing force within you. To finish the meditation, imagine that the Lotus flower fades from your awareness but continues to radiate health and harmony during your every day life. In China it is said that students who have completely mastered this exercise not only eliminate all illness in themselves, but bring health and healing to anyone they come in contact with.

As you begin to meditate it is common to have any or all of the following experiences:

1. Your mind wanders. This is quite natural and expected. Just bring yourself back to your point of focus.

2. You are unsure whether you are doing the meditation properly. You are most likely doing it right. Meditation is pretty simple to do, but more challenging to stay with.

3. You will have memories, images or thoughts that you may have not thought about in years. Just acknowledge them and bring your awareness back to your point of focus.

4. You may start to analyze yourself. Remember: this is a time for meditation, not for psychotherapy. Analyze later, meditate now.

5. You may have certain revelations. Again, acknowledge these and then bring yourself back to your point of focus.

6. A body part is sore or itchy. The first time you feel something in your body, just acknowledge it and bring your awareness back to your point of focus. Often, it will go away. This is caused by the meridians balancing their forces.